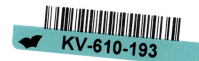
KV-610-193

# CONTENTS

# WRITING INVESTMENT PLANS AND HEALTH IMPROVEMENT PROGRAMMES

## A worce

## RADCLIFFE MEDICAL PRESS

© 1999 Roy Lilley

Radcliffe Medical Press Ltd
18 Marcham Road, Abingdon, Oxon OX14 1AA

British Library Cataloguing in Publication Data

A catalogue record for this book is available from the British Library.

ISBN 1 85775 388 7

Typeset by Advance Typesetting Ltd, Oxon.
Printed and bound by Hobbs the Printers, Totton, Hants.

# PREFACE

Like all great organisations, the NHS is evolving but it is driven by changes far more powerful than politics. Politicians come and go. The NHS outlasts them all. The real driving forces for change are to be found a million miles from Westminster. Influences that shape our daily lives and that are irresistible. The forces of technology, the refocusing of customer demand, the realisation that money for public services can only be provided in direct proportion to the numbers who work, earn and pay the taxes to make it all happen. The pressures of technology, customer demand and money.

How does that language sound to you? The words technology, customer and money. Does it seem a long way from care, patient and resources?

Technology is enabling a level of care previously not dreamed of. Increasingly, patients are seeing themselves in the role of health service customers, with the right to complain, demand services that are right first time and with the expectation that they will be treated at least as well as they are treated in their favourite high street store. Money, taxpayers' money, is not limitless and new levels of accountability and responsibility have become a permanent feature of public services.

There is a new language finding its way into healthcare, borrowed from the lexicon of business. As the NHS strives to work more effectively and use what it has more efficiently it must become more businesslike. That is not to say the NHS is a business. Businesslike is the inevitable consequence of governments, of all political flavours, realising that public services are not unique and that they should be run with the same efficiency as the private sector.

The initiatives to swing the focus of attention and modernisation onto primary care means that practitioners and others are facing sweeping changes. Changes that mean healthcare professionals and others will, for the first time, work together, in the recognition that real health is the product of wealth, social circumstances, education and life's chances.

It also means primary care will be working in a new way, a more businesslike way, adopting some of the techniques of successful business as primary care reaches for new levels of performance, accountability and quality.

Fundamental to success is careful planning. Primary Care Groups (PCGs) will now plan their future and goals around Primary Care Investment Plans – documents that seem to owe more to a background in business than they do healthcare.

PCGs will demand a new level of understanding. A knowledge of how large organisations work and a grasp of the techniques that drive them forward, will keep them efficient, solvent and effective.

If PCGs are to be businesslike then they must use the tools of business to make them work. At the foundation of every good business – chip shop or merchant bank, hotel or hospital – is a business plan. Whatever the NHS calls it and whatever language the politicians wrap it up in, business planning, in all its guises, is a fundamental skill that cannot be ignored. This workbook is about demystifying business and making planning easy. This workbook sets out to show that management is cool! There is nothing in management that is beyond the grasp of someone with common sense.

This is not a textbook or treatise, it is a workbook, a series of exercises and questions to help you clarify your thinking and it aims to 'de-puzzle' the process. This workbook is vital reading for everyone working in PCGs, playing their part and aiming for success.

PCGs parked at Levels 1 or 2, won't stay like that. Planning is an essential part of participation and moving on. Understanding the processes that health authorities use to direct PCGs means a need to understand business planning and basic management. Levels 3 and 4, with the possibility of greater self-determination, beckon. A grasp of business planning and an understanding of the fundamentals of management are two essential rungs on the ladder of progress.

Roy Lilley
*February 1999*

# ABOUT THE AUTHOR

**Roy Lilley** is a visiting fellow at the Management School, Imperial College London. He is a writer and broadcaster on health and social issues and has published over a dozen books on health, health service management and related topics.

He is the author of the original, best selling, *PCG Tool Kit* (now up-dated in its second edition), a workbook for professionals working and developing Primary Care Groups, and *The PCG Team Builder*, a workbook to help PCGs develop and work as a team.

A former businessman, he brings an understanding of the world of business, to over 20 years of work and service in the NHS and local government.

He works across the NHS and with PCGs, to help them with the challenges of modern management. He is an enthusiast for radical policies that address the real needs of patients, professionals and the communities they serve.

Without the help of dedicated NHS and local authority professionals, who have been prepared to spend their time in sharing their ideas and solutions to problems, this workbook would not have been possible. Out of a sense of admiration for the way they juggle resources, conjure solutions and walk the tightrope of policy, this workbook is dedicated to them.

We take for granted the skills of the managers who run our public services. Indeed, politicians of all political parties have made it a sport to knock them and belittle their contribution. They do so at their peril. In over 30 years of business, I remain convinced the best managers are to be found at the top of our great public services. They work under the most enormous pressure and produce results that, did they not do it so regularly, would be thought of as miracles!

And, to the best planner of the use of resources I know, EL.

# MAKING THIS BOOK WORK FOR YOU

Don't read this workbook! You won't hear many authors say they don't want you to read their book! Seriously, it is not the idea. The trick, right now, is to get a feel for the book and how it works. Flick through the pages. Scribble some notes in the margins. Fold down the corners of the pages that really interest you. Tear some pages out. Yup, I give you permission to treat the book badly!

You have bought a workbook and I want you to make it *work* for you. Some of the stuff will be too easy and other bits should make you think. The idea is to end up with the knowledge and confidence to produce a plan to be proud of. A document that jumps off the page and says '*Wow*'! A document that makes other people say '*Wow, I wish I could do that*!'

All the management toffs will tell you it's difficult. It's not! Management is clear thinking, planning and commonsense. It is also very cool!

So, make yourself a cup of coffee, sit down and flip through the book. Get a feel for the sections and the layout. I'll wait right here for you!

## Welcome back!

You will have come across some strange stuff like this:

There are a number of **Think Boxes** that are there to get the juices flowing and to get you thinking outside the box and looking at the issues from a different dimension.

There are **Hazard Warnings** that are there to point out some tricky issues, or traps not to fall into.

The **Tips** are short cuts and quick fixes to get to the answer faster.

The **Exercises** are there for you to address the issues in the context of where you work and what your task is, regardless of your profession or seniority in the organisation. When you've finished the exercises you should end up with something that looks like a business plan. Some of the exercises are there to make you think or assemble some of the elements that are needed in the plan. This is not a 'right' or 'wrong' workbook – it asks the questions in the context of the issues so you won't overlook an important topic or duck some of the tricky ones. And, and this is the important bit, figure out the best way forward for your plan.

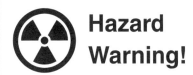

# Hazard Warning!

**Primary care investment planning in one hour! You must be joking …**

*'Planning in one hour! You must be joking. Managers say it takes months to produce a plan – how am I, with no experience, expected to do it in one hour?'*

Yup, we can hear you say it. Is this workbook a rip-off? Are we promising something you can't do? Have you got good cause to take the book back to the shop and swap it for something useful on rose growing or body piercing?

The first point to make is, don't listen to deadhead managers, or gurus who speak gobbledegook and want to make a mystery out of planning. Of course you can write a plan in an hour. It might take a bit longer to assemble the detail you need to put into the plan. You might have to take some time, learning what goes into a plan and why. You may have to hang around for colleagues to come up with the information you need to compile the detail. You may have to reserve a bit of thinking time, to clarify your mind and the thoughts of the people you are working with. But writing a plan is easy.

Follow the steps and exercises in the workbook and you will have got together all the stuff you need to produce a *'Wow'* investment plan and still be home in time for tea!

If you and your team are very new to this type of planning, the set of exercises in the introduction is designed to get you in the mood and get the juices flowing. To get you thinking about the issues and to crystallise your thoughts. The exercises can be done alone or they can be done in pairs, or in a team.

Working together on the exercises will help promote a sense of 'team' and ownership. You may like to use them in conjunction with a fabulous book called *The PCG Team Builder*, published by Radcliffe and written by some brilliant writers that modesty forbids me identifying …

In fact, if you cut out the next page of the book and send it to Radcliffe you can buy any of the books in the PCG range at a discount.

If you are a seasoned planner, you can skip these pages. But, hold on, if you are a seasoned planner, what did you buy this book for? Send off for the other ones!

# INTRODUCTION: WHAT DO YOU WANT TO DO?

If you want to, you can launch straight into the 'how to write the Primary Care Investment Programme (PCIP)' chunk of the book. It's your book, no one can stop you!

However...

...if you are new to the planning game or are working with new colleagues on PCIPs for the first time, spend a while looking through this first section. It introduces some of the fundamentals and tries to help you look beyond planning and think about why we do it and its impact on the organisation.

Essentially a PCIP is a business plan. PCGs are big complex businesses – as you are destined to find out. Having a thorough understanding of how planning processes work might come in useful one day!

 Take a break, have a coffee, flip through the pages and decide if the next section is for you and your colleagues...

## Exercise

 What makes a good plan?

Draw a line down the middle of this box. On the left-hand side write five reasons why planning may not be a good idea. Things such as *too restrictive* and the like. On the other side of the line write five reasons why planning is a good idea, knowing *where you are* and so on.

*If you are working with others, split the group into two and use two flip charts instead of this page to do the same exercise.*

Finished? Now, rip the page out of the book and pin it on the wall. When you are assembling your plan refer to it so you can maximise the benefits of planning and minimise the 'dis-benefits'.

## What can you expect a plan to do for you ?

A good plan will answer the three fundamental **find outs**:

1 **find out** where you are now

2 **find out** where you want to end up

3 **find out** how to cover the ground between points 1 and 2.

If you are planning in a group, here are the top 10 reasons for planning.

1 Enables everyone to know where the starting point is.

2 Focuses everyone's attention and gathers thoughts and ideas.

3 Helps everyone understand what the organisation is trying to achieve.

4 Brings everyone together and helps promote teamworking.

5 Generates agreement on what the group should be trying to do.

6 Exposes what the organisation is good at, what it is not good at, what it should be taking advantage of, and what it should be worrying about. *In the language of the management guru gobbledegook it is called a SWOT analysis. SWOT stands for Strengths, Weaknesses, Opportunities and Threats.*

7 Gives the organisation a sense of purpose and discipline.

8 Creates a 'map of the journey'.

9 Provides benchmarks on the way to see how you are doing.

10 Makes the case for funding the project or venture.

## Exercise

 *Do this exercise on your own, or better still with the group you will be working with.*

There are six basic steps to take into account:

1  where you are now

2  what the current activities are

3  strengths, weaknesses, opportunities, threats – of and to the plan

4  what your aim is

5  what your objectives are

6  how you will implement the plan. (*In guru speak that is sometimes referred to as 'roll-out.'*)

In not more than three words for each heading, write down your kneejerk response to each question. Compare your answers with others working with you on the project. Discuss the impressions that you have and develop an action plan to address the issues.

The 'two box' technique to help you think outside the box...

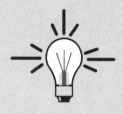

**THINK BOX**

Be honest! Did you find that last exercise difficult? If you did, try this one to help clarify your thinking about where you are starting from. If you are not being honest, don't bother with the rest of the workbook. Go and find something useful to do, like polishing the cat's eyes on the M6!

| *What services do you offer now?* | *Who are they for?* |
|---|---|
| | |

| *Over the past five years the following has changed* | *The reasons for change are* |
|---|---|
| | |

See, it's easy, just take your time and with some commonsense you can order your thoughts and start the foundation of a good plan. Use this 'two box' technique to address the other questions.

Who needs a guru?

## Exercise

 A big part of successful *planning for change* is about understanding the reasons for change and what it might achieve.

PCGs are bringing a radical change to the way in which primary care works. Those changes are impacting in a number of ways. Here are four questions for you to consider and write down your answers. *If you are working with a group, have each individual answer the questions and then compare your answers with each other.*

1 PCGs will benefit patients because…

2 PCGs will be good for the practice I work in because…

3 PCGs will help deliver national health improvement targets because…

4 PCGs will help us to focus on local issues because…

## Exercise

 Now do the mirror exercise, i.e. the reverse of the last exercise.

PCGs are bringing a radical change to the way in which primary care works. Those changes are impacting in a number of ways. Here are four questions for you to consider and write down your answers. *If you are working with a group, have each individual answer the questions and then compare your answers with each other.*

1 PCGs will be bad for patients because...

2 PCGs will be no good for the practice I work in because...

3 PCGs will struggle to deliver national health improvement targets because...

4 PCGs will play no part in helping us to focus on local issues because...

Now take the time to compare the answers to the two groups of questions. Can you see what's happening? You are starting to get a feel for the strengths and weaknesses involved in the PCG structure. More significantly, you can start to see what you need to do to plan around the weaknesses and build on your strengths.

## Will you or won't you?

---

## Exercise

Try the same technique with the following three questions. It is important to do the wills and the won'ts, so don't cheat.

1 PCGs will/won't improve the quality of care because...

2 PCGs will/won't improve patient satisfaction because...

3 PCGs will/won't have sufficient funding to work effectively because...

---

Now you've got that straight in your mind you know what you need to put into your plan to avoid the pit falls.

## This is a compass exercise or, in other words, where the *#$!@ are we now?

List the Top 10 most demanding things your PCG board will have to do *and* have a stab at what they are likely to cost. For the purpose of the exercise take 'demanding' to mean something that incurs high costs or a lot of professional time.

| *Demanding things we will have to do* | *Rough cost (yearly)* |
|---|---|
| 1 | |
| 2 | |
| 3 | |
| 4 | |
| 5 | |
| 6 | |
| 7 | |
| 8 | |
| 9 | |
| 10 | |

Done? Next step, take the costs under each heading and estimate the proportion of the total annual budget it takes up.

| *Cost heading* | *Proportion of cost* |
|---|---|
| | |
| | |
| | |
| | |
| | |
| | |

What's the point of all this? The idea is to give you a feel for the numbers involved and a sense of proportion. It is also a bit of an eye opener to see how much it costs to have a highly paid community nurse sitting in a committee. Oh, didn't you include that? Well...

## No point in being in a PCG if there aren't some tangible benefits. Let's look for some!

The purpose of this exercise is to think about what things could be done better and to prepare ourselves for including them as part of our future planning. Add to the list if you want to!

| Things we do | Could we do it any better? (Score 1 if you don't think you could and up to 5 if you see an opportunity) | What do we have to do to do it better? |
|---|---|---|
| 1 Completing items of service claims | | |
| 2 Writing prescriptions | | |
| 3 Handling repeat prescriptions | | |
| 4 Handling correspondence | | |
| 5 Appointment system | | |
| 6 On call rotas | | |
| 7 Handling patient complaints | | |
| 8 | | |
| 9 | | |
| 10 | | |

How high was the total score? Come on now, tell the truth! If you're not honest, we'll send you off to comb the lawn...

## How prepared are you for the brave new world of running a PCG?

If you are working alone, use the following headings to prompt some honest thoughts about where you are – use a 1 to 5 scoring system and see where you need to do some work!

If you are using the exercise for a team or group, give them 15 minutes to think about the questions and to jot down some answers. Then bring them into a discussion and use a flip chart to summarise their answers. This is another one of those SWOT jobs, pointing up your internal strengths and weaknesses.

## Exercise

*Personnel issues*

1 Do all staff in the practices have job descriptions?
2 Are staff regularly appraised?
3 Is there a variation between practices?
4 Does it produce conflict?

*Communication*

1 Do all practices in the PCG have regular practice meetings?
2 Are the meetings effective at cascading communication – how do you know?
3 How will you ensure all staff across the PCG know what is going on?

*Finance*

1 Is all income routinely monitored in all practices?
2 Do you personally understand the accounting system?
3 Do all practices in the PCG regularly produce monthly management accounts?
4 Is expenditure in all the practices routinely monitored?
5 Does everyone use the same system – are there anomalies?
6 If budgets, even nominal budgets, are cascaded, how can you protect against careless overspending?

## Be a swot and do another SWOT exercise!

This time the idea is to look outside at what the gurus call external boundaries. That's jargon speak for what could happen, from outside, to screw up what we're doing. More jargon speak is impact analysis. See, management is easy if you know the words! Take five years as a reasonable time envelope.

| *External factor* | *Possible impact* |
| --- | --- |
|  |  |

## A mission to succeed

This is the 'vision thing'. Organisations work better when everyone knows what they are supposed to be doing. One of the ways of galvanising those thoughts and directing the energy is to have a mission statement. They don't have to be wordy or pompous, or too long. Just a simple statement of what the organisation is trying to do and how it will go about doing it. Put another way, the organisation's purpose.

The purpose needs to be a shared direction, something all the staff believe in and respect. A simple statement of aims or values can unite organisations around a common purpose.

Take some time to think about a mission statement and include it in your plan.

Here's a start:

The purpose of our PCG is ..............(*by/how*)......... to ....... (*what you want to do*) .............. that ........... (*your unique objective*) ........ by .......... (*how you intend to achieve it*) ...............

Here is an example:

> 'The Sunny Town PCG aims to use all of its resources and the skills and talents of every one working here to provide easily accessible health services that respond to people's needs, by listening to what patients want and putting them first.'

Write your's here:

## The missing bits

Now you are a plan with a mission, what new skills does the PCG need to deliver it?

| *What new skills do we need?* | *How will we get them?* |
| --- | --- |
| | |

## Agree or disagree?

This is an exercise to use at the end of a planning session, designed for the team to compare their thoughts and perceptions. Ask the team to complete the questionnaire and then collect the results (no names needed) and see if there are any real differences in results. If there are, use them as discussion points.

| Statement | Perception | | | | |
|---|---|---|---|---|---|
| | Agree | | | Don't agree | |
| | 5 | 4 | 3 | 2 | 1 |
| 1  I am much clearer about what is and isn't important | | | | | |
| 2  It focused my attention on patients | | | | | |
| 3  I have a better understanding of resource issues | | | | | |
| 4  The mission is something that I can use to guide my thinking about what is important | | | | | |
| 5  The process concentrated my thoughts | | | | | |
| 6  We were able to work as a team | | | | | |
| 7  The SWOT stuff made things a lot clearer for me | | | | | |
| 8  The NHS has no place for business, and planning is a distraction from looking after patients | | | | | |
| 9  It helped me to agree with colleagues and see their point of view | | | | | |
| 10  We now have a 'map' to set us off in the right direction | | | | | |
| 11  We can make a much better case for resources | | | | | |
| 12  We can measure our progress | | | | | |

## Think about the future?

Plans are not just for the here and now, they are for the future too. Even if you are planning for a short time span, what is likely to turn up from around the corner – the future – is worth a thought. If you have a rigid plan that cannot accommodate unexpected change or has given no thought to what the future looks like, then sorry to disappoint you, 'cause it ain't no plan!

## Think five years from now. What services will we be offering?

| What new services might we be offering in five years time? | Why do you think that? |
| --- | --- |
| | |

And, let's do the mirror exercise.

| What services might we not be offering in five years time? | Why do you think that? |
| --- | --- |
| | |

## The good, the bad and the ugly!

Let's do a round up exercise to pull together our SWOT.

| What are we not so good at? | What have we got to do to fix it? | What's our objective? | Who's going to do it and by when? |
| --- | --- | --- | --- |
|  |  |  |  |

| What are we good at? | How can we use it to our advantage? | What's our objective? | Who's going to do it and by when? |
| --- | --- | --- | --- |
|  |  |  |  |

| What are the opportunities open to us? | How can you be sure? | What's our objective? | Who's going to do it and by when? |
| --- | --- | --- | --- |
|  |  |  |  |

| What's likely to threaten us? | What can we do to reduce the threat? | What's our objective? | Who's going to do it and by when? |
| --- | --- | --- | --- |
|  |  |  |  |

Note the last column in each row – who's gonna do it and by when – very important to have what the gurus call *controlled, measured outcome objectives*.

## No one plans to fail they simply fail to plan

A plan is a road map, a set of signposts to follow, to reach a destination. The plan also makes those undertaking the journey think about whether the journey is necessary or likely to be completed successfully.

Put another way: a plan is a management tool that can help define the future and sort out what is likely to be friendly fire and what isn't. It should quantify what can and can't be reasonably done, as well as strike the balance between what the organisation wants to achieve and what it can't achieve over a fixed time period.

**A plan is not a document for dreamers or a wish list of how it could be. It is a realistic document that the organisation is prepared to be measured against.**

A plan is not written on a tablet of stone, it is a working document that can be reviewed and added to along the way. The plan will provide the information that is required now, to help make the decisions you will face tomorrow.

## THINK BOX

Planning is not demanding, but it is painstaking. Assembling the detail is important and will take time and must be as accurate as you can make it. If you can do simple arithmetic and have a standard calculator, you are on your way. But, what are the pressures on your time and, more importantly, the pressures on the time of the people you will need to go to, to assemble the information for the plan. Writing a plan takes an hour, assembling the details takes... Who knows how long it takes. So, be sure you leave yourself time. Don't agree to silly deadlines and be realistic.

# The Primary Care Investment Plan

# SECTION 1

## You've got to do one, so what is it?

### Primary Care Investment Plans (PCIPs) explained

Here are the key starting points.

Plans cover a three year cycle, so the first ones will run from 1999 to 2002. Time scales are tight. You will have needed a discussion document ready by mid-January 1999 to cover 1999–2000. A finalised plan to reflect the 1999–2000 budget and to cover the two further years to 2001–02, needs to be ready by the end of September 1999. So what are you waiting for!

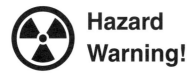 **Hazard Warning!**

This is a very tight time scale and, very often, the job has to be done by people who have a 'day job'. At Levels 1 and 2 the instinctive thing to do is to let the host health authority find someone to get on with the job. BAD IDEA. Don't do that. It is essential that the PCG signs up to the PCIP, is comfortable with what is in it, learns how to do it for themselves and feels able to deliver it.

## What goes in this wretched thing, anyway?

Your plan must summarise how you intend to deal with the following nine issues:

1 protecting the current expenditure in General Medical Services (GMS) and wider primary care provision

2 protecting current cost-effective services for patients

3 providing a planning tool for further improvement

4 addressing issues of equity of access

5 focusing on quality and how to improve it

6 linking with the local Health Improvement Programme

7 ensuring GP premises are suitable

8 linking with partners for the integration of strategies, such as trusts and social services

9 linking to the NHS IM&T strategy.

All agreed with the health authority...

 Easy! Put the kettle on...

# Wot about the money!

PCGs will operate with two budgets – management cost allocation and a unified budget.

There is £22 million in the system for PCG preparatory costs in the shadow year. This means about £55 000 for the average PCG. You can use the money for:

admin, training, support staff and office kit, GP locum costs and payments to support the involvement of GPs and nurses.

It is doubtful whether you could get away with a PCG training course in Bermuda – but it's worth a try…

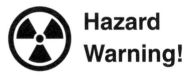 **Hazard Warning!**

Unified budgets means there's no where to go when you run out of cash. Make a mental note to find out about risk management strategies (*see PCG Tool Kit*, Second edition).

**Management cost allocations** will cover the running cost of managing the PCG. In the first year you can expect it to be worth no more than £300 000 for the average PCG in 1999/2000. There is some other cash in the system for the preparatory year, to pay for set-up training and so on.

The **unified budget** is a bit more complicated. This is a major change in the way in which the NHS is funded. From All-fools Day, 1999 (sorry couldn't resist that!), the cash-limited GMS budget, the prescribing budget and the hospital and community health services budget (HCHS) are combined into one great pile of money that will find its way to you via the health authority. The allocations are based on a national weighted capitation formula. Once it reaches the health authority, they have to allocate it to the PCGs in their area. But, first they can top slice the cash under the following headings:

- health authority functions such as public health

- joint commissioning, where two or more PCGs agree to work collaboratively on a project

- an agreed amount as a risk management reserve.

…then, if there is any left (ho, ho).

The health authority gives the PCG an allocation based on:

• the national formula

• plus, the current baseline cost of any policy they might dream up to bring all PCGs roughly in line.

Health authorities have a lot of power here, but they are obliged to develop policies for allocations that are transparent and fair and are the result of discussion with GPs and NHS trusts.

Trusts are brought into the discussions because they get paid for doing work that GPs send them. If there is a change in GP funding, referral patterns can change and trusts could be in trouble.

## Exercise

How have current arrangements impacted on referral patterns in your area? Have there been any dramatic changes? Are PCGs designed to bring about major change or are they an instrument for stability and cost management?

In the above terms list the benefits and 'dis-benefits' of PCGs. What needs to be done to impact on the 'dis-benefits'?

And, by the way…

The document must be inclusive, you need to collect the views of practices, the public, professional forums, user groups and Uncle Tom Cobley.

## Exercise

 Given the tight time scales devise a consultation model to take into account the views of all groups with a legitimate interest.

You might want to start by thinking '*who has a legitimate interest?*'

## Let's have a look at the issues in more detail and see what needs to go into the plan. There are eleven elements

### Element 1 Calculate the baseline requirement for GMS infrastructure support

It is easy to take for granted items funded from the GMS cash-limited budget. Indeed, it is easy to take the whole process for granted. Some folk find the topic of GMS a yawn. Now is the time to get a grip! Be honest, how much attention have you paid to the GMS budget? Do you really understand it? If your answer is anything but '*I understand it perfectly, thank you*', then you're probably looking down the double barrels of trouble and grief!

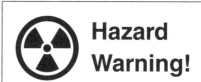

**Hazard Warning!**

Get this wrong and you are probably looking down the double barrels of trouble and grief!

You need a friend! Who do you know who can explain the detail to you? Be sure to find out because the calculations that emerge this year, could provide the foundation for future calculations. So, they've got to be right. The whole financial foundation might be wrong and, more importantly, very difficult to correct.

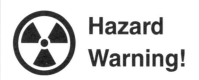

**Hazard Warning!**

The amount allocated to the PCG as the guaranteed level of expenditure is known as the floor. A PCG may wish to spend more than the 'floor' on cost improvements in PCG infrastructure. But beware, you'll have to make a good case because your PCG plans will have to compete with other PCG funding priorities.

### Exercise

GMS is calculated on the basis of returns made by GPs and practices and allocations are made via the health authority from the centre. Recheck the calculations to ensure they are correct.

## Element 2  The PCG's plans for additional GMS investment

Although the headline implies that only new investments should be added, in fact, existing commitments have to be included here as well.

These commitments might include:

• commitments to premises, such as cost rents, local authority economic rents, improvement grants and lease buy-outs

• IT capital investment or leasing (even if funding is managed by the health authority).

At the planning stage it is OK to include plans that are aspirational as well as agreed commitments. However, when the final plan is agreed with the health authority, only the *agreed* commitments for the first year of the plan should be included.

Investment in practice staff, computing, premises developments, IT and developments related to the Health Improvement Programmes (of which, more later) should be included.

This is important, don't dismiss it. You can seldom do new things without 'new people' and new places to do it.

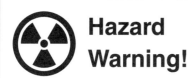 **Hazard Warning!** GMS infrastructure funds become available, locally, when GPs opt to switch from cost rent to notional rent, complete an improvement grant, or IT investment. Any such funds, while forming part of the GMS floor at health authority level, can be re-deployed, flexibly, between PCGs in line with their development needs, as set out in the PCG investment plan.

## Exercise

 Audit the improvements you have in mind in the context of extra staff, premises improvement and IT.

Element 3 Proposals for new investment in GMS infrastructure to be financed from the health authority's out-of-hours development fund of the national GMS non cash-limited budget

Items under this heading are the responsibility of the health authority. However, you have the key!

The health authority has to show 'value for money' for the plans and who better to advise on value for money? You won't need three guesses!

## Exercise

Value for money (VFM) can be evaluated in several ways. VFM over a long term, VFM evaluated against current ways of doing things, VFM in the sense of stopping doing something one way and starting to do it in another. VFM is not about cheapest or fastest. The key is the evaluation of the word 'value' in the context of the plan.

Value may mean paying more in the short term, in order to gain value in the longer term.

In a great book written by a friend – John Marriotti, *Shape Shifters* (published by VNR) – John describes value for money as a pentangle, made up of quality, service, cost, speed and innovation.

He draws it like this:

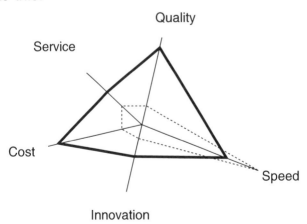

As you can see, there is a thick black line that joins the key components. The closer the line is to the title, the more important it is. This model describes a

service that needs to be fast, not specially innovative, cheap to acquire, with a high level of quality and without much service required to back it up. The dotted line describes something quite different.

This is a simple way to get your head the right way round when evaluating what VFM means in your context.

Draw a pentangle to evaluate VFM on three projects:

• meals-on-wheels services for the housebound elderly

• a clinic for adults, in employment, suffering depression

• the purchase of a new photocopying machine for the surgery.

See how the shapes change?

Use the evaluation pentangle for your plans. Remember, the idea is not to create diagrams, it is to create VFM.

## Element 4  A stocktake of existing practice-based services

In technical terms these are the services provided under HSG (96)31, PMS arrangements and Section 36 GMS local developed schemes!

Ugh! Forget the gookspeak. The idea is to establish the baseline of services not so that someone can take a pace back and say 'what wonderful services we offer'. It is so the health authority can get an idea of the ongoing financial picture, and, in the longer run, to spot where any service gaps may emerge.

So, the trick here is to be thorough. This is not a beauty competition. List everything, good and bad – it will pay off in the long run.

## Exercise

Go do it, make the audit!

## Element 5 Plans for new practice-based services

Now, this is getting much more interesting. New stuff, new ideas, all very exciting.

Now is the time to realise that PCGs are not just about your practice, they are about everyone in the group. Finding out what they all want to do, avoiding duplication and focusing on what really needs to be done is not so easy.

Some practices are likely to be mortified if they see their dreams trashed. Whadareyergonnado!

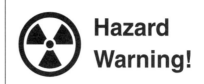

**Hazard Warning!**

This is where you must include proposals for new personal medical services pilots and any new Section 36 schemes.

Well, all you can do is to take it step by step.

Set some time limits for practices to present their schemes. Make it clear there is a cut off date and they must deliver on time. Allow time for a thorough evaluation of what they want to do and allow even more time to allow for some friendly persuasion and arm twisting.

In management jargon this comes under the heading of a 'health needs assessment'. Health authorities are obliged to make regular reviews of the health of the local population and to spot what needs to be improved. They will have some policy aims and objectives to deal with gaps in the service and ways of monitoring their progress.

The health authority will be drawing a little map called an SND map. It's got nothing to do with a Scottish political party and stands for supply, need, demand. It will look like this:

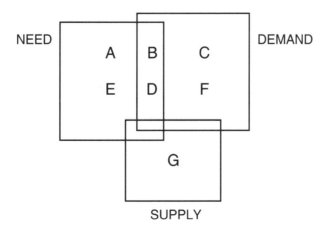

Here's the A, B and C of how it works.

A  Unknown and therefore unmet areas of need where there is a chance to do some good stuff, such as in non-insulin dependent diabetes or blood pressure problems in men of working age.

B  Known unmet demand, such as waiting lists.

C  Justifiable unmet demand, such as tattoo removal (Yup, I know there can sometimes be a social need for this tattoo removal).

D  This is 'happy land' where demand is met.

E  Services in the health promotion category that are good for patients but also have organisational or demand management pluses for the health authority, such as clinics to help people lose weight.

F  Services that are there to meet demand, not need. This includes services such as in-hospital surgery that could be done as a day case.

G  Services that no one uses.

So, the more services that fall into sector D the better. Shifting investment from sector G might enable better use of the money in sector B.

See management is easy – it's all about drawing pictures! Makes things clearer though, doesn't it? And it helps to justify decisions.

## Exercise

 Look at the list of services offered by your practice. Make an SND map. How would you shuffle the services?

Compare a list of services practice by practice. Make SND maps of them all and compare them. What are the obvious differences? What needs to be changed?

# Exercise

 One of the keys to good evaluation, that even people disappointed by the outcome might agree with, is to use a system that is transparent and fair.

Devise a list of key points against which you could evaluate proposals. The list might include:

- VFM

- fills an unmet need

- innovative and worth considering as a trial for evaluation

- 

- 

- 

- 

Don't overcomplicate the list by making it too long and try and keep the evaluation points simple. That way they are difficult for the wicked to unpick.

## Element 6  A review of the local primary care workforce

Can't get the staff, eh? I wonder why! There are all kinds of statistics about staffing that could fill this book twice over. And none of them are good news.

Don't say it to nurses but the statistics show that they're getting older. A very significant proportion of them are coming up to retirement age and training the new ones is taking longer. Not only that, because of competition in the jobs market, fewer youngsters are seeing nursing as a career prospect.

It's the same with doctors. About one-third of the places on vocational courses to become GPs are empty. Young doctors seem to like the idea of swishing down a hospital corridor in a white coat, but not the idea of driving around some god-forsaken part of 'down-town' in the dead of night, trying to make a house call.

Some of the professions allied to medicine seem to be facing extinction – physiotherapy, for example, is facing its own recruitment difficulty.

This is serious stuff and the Gods of Whitehall are worried. Pay is partly an issue but there are so many other factors, it makes you wonder what the solutions really are.

For your PCG, so-called workforce planning is a serious topic. We need to start by finding out where you are now.

List:

• the number and types of doctors
• the numbers and types of nurses employed by the practices
• support clinical staff
• management staff.

Next, identify the problems:

• recruitment
• retention
• skill mix
• training needs.

# Exercise

 Use the results of the previous analysis to develop objectives and plans to address training needs and to address retention and recruitment problems in key areas.

Consider how you could present the PCG in the most attractive light to attract new staff.

Consider devising a recruitment strategy for the PCG as a whole rather than leaving it to individual practices.

What are the advantages and disadvantages of this approach?

## Element 7  Community nursing

Are you ready for this?

PCGs will assume more and more responsibility for the delivery of total community care. Nursing plays a pivotal role and is part of government strategy to shift care from the secondary sector to the primary sector.

This element will probably be part of your future plans for the PCG, to develop services. Well, there's no point in developing great ideas if you don't have the people to make them a reality.

Nurse-led services, such as for patients with diabetes or asthma, are becoming almost standard. Can you find the nurses to do it? And, the job doesn't stop with finding them. They will need continuing professional development and training.

Looking across the whole landscape of healthcare, nurse-led rapid response teams and home support services can have a real impact on waiting lists by supporting earlier discharge from hospital. Generally, nurses working closely with social services can make a real difference. Practice nurses, taking their own case work, are popular with patients, speed access to services and help GPs.

So, what services are you planning that involve nursing?

## Exercise

 Audit current services and service development plans. What is the nurse impact? Develop recruitment and training strategies to underpin the developments.

With particular reference to nurses working with social services, devise a training approach to make it easier for the two to work together.

## Element 8 Proposals for the deployment of former fundholders' savings

Did I hear you say 'what savings?' Such cynicism in one so young!

Fundholders coming out of the scheme at the end of 1998–99 will have the costs of their disestablishment met from their savings. After that, what happens to their savings is a matter for negotiation between them, the PCG and the health authority.

Subject to agreement, fundholders can spend the money on schemes that benefit their patients and, subject to it fitting in with the PCIP, on their premises.

However, unlike fundholding, there is no automatic right to roll-over. Anything not spent in year one gets pinched by the PCG!

When you've tiptoed around all this lot, the PCIP should incorporate the 'savings plans' agreed between the PCG and the former fundholders, for the use of the balance of the inherited savings after the fund has been closed.

If the fundholders and the PCG can't agree, the plan must show how the fundholders themselves intend to use their guaranteed savings entitlements.

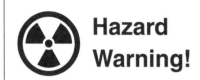 **Hazard Warning!**

Agreement on how fundholder savings are used has to be arrived at by October 1999.

If agreement can't be reached the savings are put in the bank and the fundholder gets 25% of the cash each year (or £25 000, whichever is the lower) for four years.

The main issue here is not to force people down one road or another, it's about showing where the money will be spent.

## Exercise

What is the percentage of fundholders to non-fundholders in your PCG?

How is this likely to impact on the medium-term investment strategy for your PCG?

## Element 9 The PCG practice incentive scheme

Here's some good news, ten steps to paradise.

Under what is called 'incentive arrangements', there are ten principles that are the baseline for the PCG to put incentive arrangements in place.

1 Reward PCGs who have taken on responsibility and done it in a clinically and cost-effective manner.

2 Rewards are made at the level at which the decisions are made.

3 Reward value for money high-quality care.

4 Fits in with national and other initiatives and rewards improvements in access and equity.

5 Is balanced between PCG overall and practice-based improvement.

6 Simple to operate.

7 Be motivational.

8 Reward good practices even if the PCG is poor.

9 Allow for year-on-year performance.

10 Incentivise good performers to help poor performers.

Further incentives can include a prescribing incentive scheme to keep costs down.

### In practical terms what does it all mean?

If a practice gets lucky and benefits from windfall savings, all bets are off and the money goes to the PCG for redistribution. However, if they are clever boys and girls and they create savings through being good at what they do, they get to keep the first £10 000. After that it all gets a bit complex and will, no doubt, become a new battle ground for the negotiators. In simple terms, the next £70 000 of practice savings is split 50/50 with the practice and the PCG. Savings over £80 000 are up for discussion.

A couple of important points. The PCG's first duty is to spend its share of savings on bailing out overspenders and a practice cannot (without the agreement of the health authority), accumulate its share of the savings to save up for some mega, gold-plated idea.

So you've got your savings, what can you spend the money on? Take the whole of the practice to the pub for a good night out? A week in Bali for the chairman and his wife? Sorry, no!

Here's the list:

- material or equipment for treating patients, such as defibrillators, nebulisers and bits of kit and the associated consumables like that
- lifestyle counsellors for providing advice on how to give up smoking, or get thin, or come off the booze
- kit for the practice, such as air-conditioning, vending machines and anything that makes the place more comfortable or convenient for patients and staff
- computers and software
- non-recurring staff costs
- anything to improve prescribing
- health education kit, such as tellies, videos, leaflets and the like
- investments in premises, consistent with the PCIP.

**THINK BOX**

If this all sounds a bit like fundholding, it was you wot said it, not me!

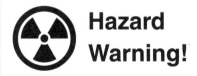

**Hazard Warning!**

Here's what you can't spend your ill-gotten gains on:

services or kit not connected with healthcare, employment costs of existing staff, purchasing land or premises, paying off loans or mortgages, drugs, medicines or appliances and hospital services.

## Exercise

Focus on the ten elements of an incentive programme. Which are likely to be the most motivating for a practice – why?

## Element 10 Achieve Modernisation Fund targets

What's the Modernisation Fund? Well, this is what the Gods of Whitehall said about it in July 1998:

'• *the Government is to create an NHS Modernisation Fund to target the extra funds for the health service on specifically planned and monitored improvements in standards of NHS buildings, plant, equipment, staff training and information technology*

• *the Government is to identify the country's best performing and most innovative hospitals, health centres and GP surgeries by designating them the title of NHS Beacons of Excellence and providing extra cash to help them spread improvement throughout the NHS.*

*The NHS Modernisation Fund will ensure that extra investment is matched to targeted improvement and reform.*

*Examples of the improvements upon which the Modernisation Fund will concentrate include:*

– *building new GP premises and refurbishing hospitals*

– *buying new, modern equipment*

– *better training for staff*

– *developing and introducing leading edge information technology.*

*The new NHS Beacons of Excellence will provide a further boost to the Government's drive to improve quality across the NHS and to spearhead its modernisation.*

*Invitations to become first-wave Beacons will be issued in October with Beacon status conferred and funded from April 1999. The Beacons will be funded from the new NHS Modernisation Fund and will serve as practical examples of the modernisation objectives that flow from the Comprehensive Spending Review.'*

OK, so now you know!

Examples of some of the areas for which NHS Beacons of Excellence could be awarded include:

- wait-free A&E services

- leading edge information technology

- pioneering quality initiatives to drive up standards of care

- outstanding programmes to reduce smoking and heart disease.

Your plan should explain the contribution your PCG will make to the achievement of the Modernisation Fund targets.

The temptation will be to pay lip service to this element of the plan. There is a huge agenda to be covered, loads of other things to do and the details surrounding the fund are, right now, far from well defined. Many commentators point out that everytime a Minister stands up and speaks about the future of the NHS, they spend the Modernisation Fund all over again!

**Take this seriously. There is serious money at stake and serious PCGs will seriously benefit!**

## So, what to do?

This is about innovation and new ideas. Don't say there isn't anything you can think of!

## Exercise

 The Modernisation Fund is something for all the members of the PCG to think about. Devise a consultation exercise to consult on ideas for bids for the Modernisation Fund.

Think about how the bids should be evaluated and which ones the PCG will support.

## Element 11 The PCG's plans for continuing professional development

Training and quality go together and the first decision must be to decide where training fits into the organisation. Is it a quality issue or is it a human resource issue? Are we training people to do what they do now better, or are we training them for the new challenges and opportunities PCGs offer?

PCGs are moving towards a public health agenda, they are not just about buying episodes of elective care.

# Exercise

- How would you select a lead person to be responsible for education and training?

- Does it have to be a doctor or nurse?

- What are the practical connections between everyday work and learning?

- How would you go about compiling a database of best practice?

- How does the approach to training change against the background of a greater emphasis on public health and closer partnerships with social services and others?

## Exercise

 Identify the links between:

- individual professional development
- practice professional development plans
- PCG strategic aims for the delivery of local services.

 PCGs can gain valuable advanced information on changes when they are consulted by health authorities on proposals for the 1999–2000 period, for new investment in practice staff, premises and computers.

# The 'what goes in' action plan

Who will do it?

By when?

Baseline calculations – this is cost formerly funded from the GMS cash-limited budget. Plus, recurrent GMS staff reimbursement and IT maintenance costs

Plans for additional GMS investment. Firm plans for the first year and 'aspirational' plans thereafter. Include commitments to existing buildings, IT capital investment or leasing for which the HA pay

Investment in staff, computing, premises development and IT

**Note:** developments should link to the local HImP and implementation of national IT strategy

Investment in infrastructure such as the out-of-hours development fund

A stock-take of existing services

Plans for any new practice-based services, including aspirational and draft plans

Review of the workforce, identifying skill-mix or recruitment problems and plans to overcome them

Developments in community and specialist nursing, such as asthma or diabetes

Proposals for the deployment of former fundholder's savings

The PCG's practice incentive scheme

An explanation of how the PCG will contribute to the Modernisation Fund targets

Plans for continuing professional development

# Health Improvement Programmes

# SECTION 2

## Just when you thought you had finished

### There is something you've got to do as well!
### Health Improvement Programmes (HImPs)

A recurring theme throughout the PCIP process is to make sure that it dovetails with another important document, the Health Improvement Programme. What is it?

 It's coffee time. Read this overview first.

**Health Improvement Programmes** or HImPs are at the heart of the Government's aim to recognise the causes of ill health and to do something about it. They are a local action plan to improve health and modernise services in the context of 'joined-up services'.

HImPs aim to:

- bring together the local NHS with local authorities and others, including the voluntary sector

- to set the strategic framework for improving health

- tackle inequalities

- develop faster, more convenient services of a consistently high standard.

In case this is starting to look like another strategic document that sits on the shelf in a manager's office, HImPs must also:

- be action focused

- set out high level objectives

- summarise the commitment of the local players to deliver these

- include measurable targets for improvement

- demonstrate how resources are to be used to improve the health and well-being of the population and to modernise the NHS.

So, no hiding place!

They must also:

- involve everyone with an interest

- engage PCGs in the strategic planning process, ensuring that the HImP is guided by the perspective and knowledge that PCGs are able to bring to bear *(See, you've got a nice mention. Very flattering, now you've got to want to be involved, haven't you?)*

- take proper account of locally determined needs

- include national priorities

- enable hospital clinicians to contribute their expertise on how best to meet local needs

- offer the opportunity for the local community and its leaders, e.g. local councillors, to influence the strategy.

So, everyone gets their say on what local health priorities should be.

## OK, that's what they are all about. How do you write one?

HImPs are new documents and no one is too sure what to do. The idea is clear enough. HImPs recognise the inextricable links that exist between health, wealth, social circumstances, education, job opportunities and the environment in which we live. Joining them together to improve our health is no bad idea. However, for services more used to working in water tight compartments, this isn't going to be easy and everyone recognises it will take time to fully develop HImPs that involve all the different local interests.

To really get into this you will have to do some extra reading. Go to bed early, with a cup of cocoa and have a thrilling time reading: *The New NHS: modern, dependable; Modernising Health and Social Services; National Priorities Guidance; Our Healthier Nation;* and *Modern Local Government: in touch with the people*. And, try and stay awake!

For the first year prioritise around building and strengthening local partnership arrangements. The first HImPs, beginning 1999–2000, are not expected to be comprehensive. They should aim to tackle a selected number of national and local issues whilst setting out the action planned to develop a fuller HImP for 2000–01, and a comprehensive HImP for the period covering 2002–03 to 2004–05

**THINK BOX**

The question here is, will PCGs be developed by the HImP or will the HImP be developed by the PCG?

### Don't start with a blank sheet of paper!

Tempting, but not the idea. HImPs should build on existing local planning and activity. So the first step is to find out what is going on in the area.

## Exercise

 Design a method of auditing current planning and activity and show how it provides the basis for your HImP.

## Here are the ingredients for a perfect HImP

### Geography

The HImP must be prepared at health authority level and cover the whole of their area. There is scope to adopt the HImP approach to more local levels, but the aim is for the HImP to cover the whole of the health authority territory. PCGs are expected to have an input into the HImP.

### Time

HImPs focus on a three year time span, rolled forward and reviewed annually. However, that is not to say that initiatives get dumped at the end of the three years. Where entrenched problems exist, a longer time frame can be envisaged. However, there must be milestones on the way so that progress can be measured and the community can see that a difference is being made.

### Involvement

Health authorities have the lead role in bringing together all the agencies and organisations that can impact on community issues. Users of local services include residents, patients and clients and the relatives, friends and carers who support them.

Organisations who provide the services include:

- PCGs

- NHS trusts

- NHS staff

- hospital clinicians

- primary care staff

- PAMs

- dentists

- pharmacists

- optometrists

- public health staff.

Others with an interest and something to offer include:

- universities

- TECs

- trade unions

- schools

- employers

- occupational health services

- business

- Health and Safety Executive.

## Exercise

 Consider how to consult with the service users and providers that have an interest in HImPs. Draw up an action plan.

## Exercise

 HImPs bring together health authorities and local authorities in a new statutory duty of partnership. Together the authorities have responsibilities that include health, health prevention, housing, crime, disorder, transport, education, environment and leisure.

Take one disease area, such as depression in women, and consider how many agencies could impact on the patient's well-being and draw up an outline action plan to involve them all.

What could you, realistically, hope to achieve?

## Record involvement

Your HImP should record who has been involved in its development and how. All partners should be encouraged to record their commitment. This approach leads to a greater community understanding of what they can expect from the HImP and helps to hold partners to account.

## Planning for future involvement

The HImP is a public document and should be available for non-English speaking communities in the appropriate languages, plus copies on tape or in braille. The document should herald issues that the next HImP document may tackle in order to give as much time as possible for communities and their leaders to become involved.

## Sharing information

The duty of partnership requires openness in sharing information needed to underpin the development of HImPs. Patient information may be used in HImPs provided it is aggregated or anonymised.

## Consultation arrangements

The ongoing nature of the HImP means that a formal consultation process should not be necessary. However, where substantial changes are envisaged, the usual consultation arrangements will apply.

### The core content:

- a needs assessment
- resource mapping
- identification of priorities
- strategies for change
- a service and financial framework.

And all the strategies to be based on evidence, clinical cost effectiveness and appropriateness.

# Exercise

Under the following five headings consider the issues that might be addressed in the HImP, the agencies involved and what outcomes could be achieved:

1  drug misuse

2  youth justice

3  crime and disorder

4  children

5  carers.

# Exercise

HImPs can be monitored under the following headings:

• health improvement

• access

• effectiveness

• efficiency

• patient and carer experience

• health outcomes.

What targets could be set to measure progress?

## Exercise

 How could transport policy be integrated into a HImP? What would be the key targets from a health perspective? For example, impact on asthma.

## Exercise

 How will you prevent the HImP becoming another report gathering dust on the shelves of the bookcase? Demonstrate how HImPs can be action focused.

## Making a start without a blank sheet of paper

For the first year don't be too ambitious! You need only aim to set a strategic framework for action on national and local priorities and an outline rolling programme for developing the full HImP. This will need to include the four *Our Healthier Nation* priority areas and action on local health inequalities.

On some issues there may already be an agreed local strategy which commands wide support. Hence, don't start with a blank piece of paper, work from what is already in place.

For other issues it may be right to plan for in-depth reviews. Set up a rolling programme that takes into account the need for work during 1999–2000 to plan the local response to the National Service Frameworks for coronary heart disease and mental health. And don't forget our old friends, Calman & Hine – ensure implementation of their existing programme.

HImPs also give us the opportunity to begin to address the commitment to modernising the NHS, announced as a result of the Comprehensive Spending Review, and show how objectives set in the National Priorities Guidance and those for the NHS Modernisation Fund will be met. See how this is starting to look like joined-up planning? The common link here is the reference to the Modernisation Fund, already playing a part in the preparation of the PCIP.

## What else?

Well, joined-up services are at the top of the agenda and that is all about service and professionals working together.

For local authorities, this represents an opportunity to engage in health improvement in its broadest sense. This comes on top of a new duty for them to promote the economic, social and environmental well-being of their areas and their proposed community planning responsibilities. This will engage the local authority corporately, across all its functions, since what determines

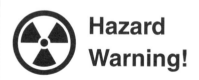

## Hazard Warning!

A new statutory duty of partnership between health authorities (including PCGs), PCTs and NHS trusts, to secure the aims and objectives of the NHS; between NHS bodies and local authorities to promote the health and well-being of their local populations.

If you don't work together – expect to go to jail!

'wellness' and good health spans the range of local authority services, such as housing, transport, education, environment and leisure.

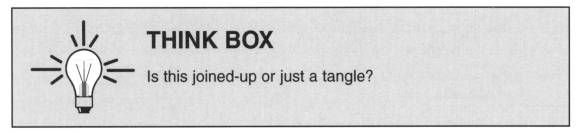

**THINK BOX**

Is this joined-up or just a tangle?

It also means local authorities will have a greater insight and a stronger voice in the early stages of NHS plans. See how joined-up this all is?

HImPs will also record, in headline form, NHS commitments on wider issues on which local authorities lead, e.g. crime and disorder and youth justice. Working together, NHS and local authority partners are expected to develop an increased understanding of each others' priorities and of the scope for effective joint action.

## What is there to build on?

There is already a good deal of joint and collaborative working going on in the public services. For example, developments in patient partnership, joint planning and working between health and social services and the voluntary sector. Plus, the early experience of HAZs, partnership working on Single Regeneration Budget schemes, and local authorities' experience of community involvement.

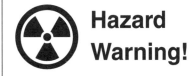 **Hazard Warning!**

HImPs are important to PCGs. They must be confident that they can influence the processes and help shape their content. Look out for consultation time scales, insist they are realistic and give you a proper opportunity to get the views of your PCG's component practices.

More detail on what goes in...

## Needs assessment

It's unlikely that one service or organisation will have all the data needed for a full needs assessment. Indeed, there is a danger of letting one service dominate the process. The assessment needs to be balanced and well judged and not skewed by the enthusiasm of one service.

Pooling the work of a number of local players, including the perspectives of PCGs and local authorities, develops a comprehensive picture (including an assessment of inequalities of access to services) and avoids duplication of effort.

## Resource mapping

Sharing baseline information and forecasts, on what resources are available. In the past, joint working has not always meant services being totally frank about resources. Ring-fenced budgets have sometimes been the incentive for services to hold back on their true position. You can hardly blame them! Joint funding was, sometimes, funding the minimum possible! Hopefully, HImPs will create more openness in the process – if only to reveal no one has any resources! Remember, the workforce is part of an organisation's resource. The best plans can flounder if there are not enough well-trained people to make them happen. The NHS has staff shortages in key areas, many of them in primary care. What's it like in local authorities? Do they have a queue of people waiting to train as social workers? Can they retain staff any better than the NHS? Partnerships are also about learning from each other – what can you learn?

## Identification of priorities for action

The priorities are driven by the national policies to be found in such tomes as the National Priorities Guidance for health and social services, *Our Healthier Nation* and other national policies and strategies driving local authorities and other partners.

...all this joins up with the local needs assessment and that joins up with...

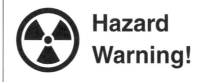 **Hazard Warning!**

Expect, over time, the National Service Frameworks and the National Institute for Clinical Excellence (NICE) guidelines to have a key role in informing local strategies. If you have something serious to say about your local strategies, get them in place early!

## Strategies for change

Objectives, targets and milestones for measurable improvement.

## We're not quite finished yet

These strategies should cover the spectrum of action on the wider determinants of health, through preventative strategies, to hospital treatment and subsequent care. HImPs should include commitments to joint action at the health and social care boundary.

And must be...

## Evidence based

It will be important that strategies are based wherever possible on sound evidence of the clinical cost effectiveness and appropriateness of interventions.

## Commitments to partner organisations

What is the NHS going to promise other public services and voluntary bodies who are part of the HImP? Because the scope of HImPs extends to improving the health and well-being of local communities in their widest sense, government thinks it is appropriate for health to record (in brief, headline terms) the NHS commitments to cross-cutting activity with, and often led by, non-NHS partner organisations.

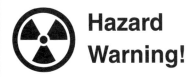 **Hazard Warning!**

Make sure you only commit yourself to what you can reasonably deliver. PCGs have a lot on their plates right now and extra items, such as cross-boundary collaboration, consume time and effort to get going. Now is not the time to be ambitious!

## Cost cutting?

Well, there's always a catch, isn't there? Two organisations working together, each with tight budgets, doesn't mean that when they come together, they will have a bigger budget. Or does it?

## Exercise

How could joint working save money? Are there operational or administrative tasks that could be combined or done cheaper? Pooling resources is not the same as merging services. Won't real savings only come from a redesign of local social and healthcare provision?

Itemise areas of possible cost saving arising from joint working.

List possible instances of increased costs that might result from joint working.

## Exercise

HImPs are important but complex documents. Keeping track of them, especially those featuring rolling programmes, is not easy.

Describe what benchmarks and milestones you could put in place to measure progress.

# Will HImPs end up on a shelf someplace or are they going to be *action documents*?

If the Gods of Whitehall have anything to do with it all this 'joined-upness' is going to make something happen. The HImP itself will set out high-level objectives and commitments. Because the accent is on implementation, making a real impact on health needs, these will need to be followed through into local operational and delivery plans, including:

* relevant strands of local authority plans

* the plans of other non-NHS partners

* the health promotion and prevention components of NHS service agreements

and PCG accountability agreements – that means you!

## Monitoring and accountability

The HImP will represent the public commitment of all the partners to improve the health and healthcare of their local communities and to provide better integrated services. An annual public report will highlight the progress against objectives and targets as the HImP is rolled forward. So, everyone will know how things are going!

### Targets what targets?

Measuring progress means targets. The HImP must identify targets for measurable improvements in health and healthcare and in reducing inequalities and specify milestones along the way. Such as:

* national priorities and guidelines, e.g. local contributions to *Our Healthier Nation* targets and national waiting list objectives

* local action to tackle local health inequalities

* improving the health of the worst off

* mapping health inequalities

* inequality in access to services.

**And**, like we would forget, the six basic principles of the 'New NHS':

- health improvement

- access

- effectiveness

- efficiency

- patient and carer experience

- health outcomes.

Just in case you are feeling slightly paranoid, with all this targeting and measuring, social services are being targeted and monitored too!

The social services White Paper will set out plans for monitoring their performance. Nothing for health to worry about – we've got enough on our minds! Local authorities do not escape and they are monitored for such good stuff as air quality, housing stock and progress on anti-poverty strategies, that in turn will contribute to health improvement targets.

The Social Exclusion Unit's Report *Bringing Britain Together: a national strategy for neighbourhood renewal* identifies valuable issues in the drive to improve local quality of life and health and is worth a read. Download it from the Central Office of Information's Website. Not wired? No chance…

A supporting *Development Pack for Health Improvement Programmes* is available, through the Regional Offices of the NHS Executive, which includes helpful detail on developing the HImP and on producing supporting strategies.

## Who's accountable for all this?

**For the NHS:**

- NHS Executive Regional Offices will hold health authorities to account for their role in the HImP (expect a new department!)

- NHS Executive Regional Offices will hold NHS trusts to account for meeting their new duty of partnership, which will be given expression through the HImP process

- 'accountability agreements with PCGs and trusts will reflect the local action needed to implement the strategic intentions in the HImP which they have helped draw up' *(these words are straight out of guidance and they are as clear as mud. The important thing is somebody will turn up and say 'whadareyerdoin?', so be prepared)*

- service agreements between health authorities, primary care trusts and NHS trusts will support the objectives of the HImP.

**At the health and social care boundary:**

Joint investment plans will need to record how they contribute to the HImP targets and milestones. NHS Executive Regional Offices, working jointly with social care regions and the government offices of the Regions, will monitor the progress achieved by health authorities and their local health partners.

# SECTION 3

## Would you know it when you saw it?

### That's all very well, but what about the real world? What does a HImP look like?

Writing a complete HImP is beyond the scope of this workbook but looking at one element of a HImP gives an insight into what the total picture might look like. So, let's look at one area where a PCG might decide to focus its attention.

The problem is, which area? Asthma, diabetes? All the 'popular' chronic diseases are begging to be the ones targeted in a HImP. Mental health is one of *Our Healthier Nation* targets and is often a Cinderella sector. Within mental health there is a condition that is probably more prevalent than asthma or diabetes, and it is depression.

Depression is the most common mental illness, is invariably treated in primary care and often involves other professionals outside health in the final treatment/management mix.

So, for the purpose of the following series of exercises, we will focus on depression. To simplify the process the exercise is practice based. To apply it to PCG planning, simply apply the exercises to all the practices that compose the PCG.

The approach could be used for any chronic illness. Just delete depression and use the technique to look at other areas!

# Exercise

How can you justify focusing on depression? This involves producing the evidence, or epidemiology. Nationally, the rate of depression in a population of 1000 patients is generally thought to be in the 30–50 region.

Establish the prevalence in your practice:

• Translate the figures into how many patients a week may present at the practice with the condition.

• What are the referral rates?

• Some illnesses make patients depressed. What is the incidence of physical illnesses presenting alongside depression (called co-morbidity)?

Government wishes to see HImPs addressing local issues and national targets. One of the targets is to reduce the incidence of suicide by 17% by 2010.

• Establish the incidence of suicide and parasuicide amongst depressed patients at your practice.

• Can you make a link between suicide and its costs in terms of A&E, bed stays, outpatient treatment, inpatient treatment, loss of working days, loss to the Benefits Agency, or other costs?

# Exercise

What are you doing for patients with depression? What are the health needs of the patients and how do you know? Improving services often involves changing the behaviour of the people providing the services. Whose behaviour needs changing? This calls for an audit...

Here are some common causes for the lack of success in treating depressed patients. Devise an audit approach that will highlight substantial variations in approach, or other inconsistencies. Discuss them with colleagues and make recommendations for changes.

- Depressed patients are often slow to reveal their true illness. How much time does the GP spend with patients who are eventually diagnosed as being depressed?

- Does co-morbidity disguise depression and delay a diagnosis?

- The side-effects of some drugs that are used to treat depression are unpleasant – do patients demonstrate poor compliance with their treatment?

- Are dosage levels too low?

- Is there any evidence that changes in dose rates or even switching to other drugs produces any better effects?

- Has the practice tried alternative therapies?

- What is the success with these therapies?

# Exercise

 If patient compliance with treatment emerges as a major problem, consider what steps you might take to improve compliance?

Consider all issues including:

- better patient information

- more modern drug therapies and the cost impact

- issues including side-effects

- the presence, or otherwise, of carer support

- 

- 

- 

- 

- 

- 

-

## Exercise

Having audited current practice, list the areas that need to be addressed and look for suitable improvement or change. Set key targets and state who is responsible for delivering the improvements.

Consider how you would conduct a rolling programme of audit to make sure any changes are implemented and are working.

## Exercise

Having had the benefit of audit, can you identify best practice? Where best practice emerges it is often possible to devise a treatment protocol that can lay the foundation of a 'care pathway'. Working with colleagues, can you establish a treatment protocol?

Does the preferred protocol lead into issues of resources or practical problems that current practice does not address? Define what needs to be changed.

## Exercise

 Consider the advice of a community pharmacist in the evaluation of present drug therapies and the potential for change.

What is the range of drugs available to treat depression and what is the likely impact in switching therapies? What are the benefits, what are the 'dis-benefits'?

## Exercise

 Nurses play an increasing role in the delivery of primary care. How are nurses engaged in the treatment of depression? Are there clear criteria for the handover of patients from the GP to the practice nurse and in the event of problems, back again?

Develop a protocol for handover.

How do community psychiatric nurses play their part? Evaluate their role and make recommendations about improving their contribution.

# Exercise

 What role is social services playing in the treatment of patients with depression? This is very important because HImPs are all about 'joined-upness' remember. Showing how other agencies can impact on a disease area is vital – working together for the benefit of the patient.

Evaluate the social services input and make recommendations about improving the service.

What partnership strategies need to be put in place?

# Exercise

 What other agencies play a part in the lives of people suffering depression and may have an impact on the 'wellness' of a patient?

Make a list. Here's a few to start:

- housing

- employment

- employers

- Benefits Agency

- Relate

- Alcoholics Anonymous

- education

- 

- 

- 

- 

- 

- 

- 

- 

Consider the impact of these agencies and organisations. Develop a strategy for involving them in a way that helps patients without stigmatising them.

# Exercise

 There may come a time when a patient might be better treated in secondary care. Evaluate the criteria for urgent and non-urgent referral. Is the practice consistent in its approach or are there variations? Why?

What is the cost of referral? Can it be reduced?

Work with colleagues to develop a set of criteria for referral.

# Exercise

 Where can you establish 'best practice' for the treatment of patients with depression?

Make a list of likely organisations and contact them for best practice guidelines.

How does 'best practice' compare with your practice?

OK, that's it, time for a coffee!

By working through these exercises you now have a very good understanding of the strengths and weaknesses of the services you offer to patients with depression. It is far from definitive but it will be enough for you to see what is good about the service and what could be improved.

It is now possible for you to build on your work and use it as one element of a HImP. Using the opportunity of the HImP to focus attention and resources on one part of your services. A part that can be monitored and audited again to watch you progress and for you to see how you are working, with others, to bring about change.

By integrating the HImP with the PCIP (this is starting to look like the recipe for alphabet soup!) you can see how joined-up services might just work!

All very joined-up!

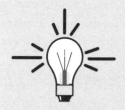

**THINK BOX**

Is it really very joined-up or is it too complex? Will HImPs and PCIPs really be action documents or will they end up like so many other strategic documents in the public sector...?

Are they stepping stones for change or a managerial millstone to be lifted up once a year?

# New lamps for old!

Primary Care Investment Plans are a product of the Department of Health's drive to find new words for old phrases. At another time, in the history of the NHS, a Primary Care Investment Plan might have been called a Primary Care Business Plan.

Government is at pains to decouple from the market-led reforms of the 1990s and with it the language of business that underpinned them. The early White Papers and guidance that signalled Labour's 're-building' of the NHS avoided words that linked them with the past. There was no mention of 'Boards' or 'Directors'. In subsequent guidance and circulars the language of business has re-emerged.

Raising this issue is to make no other point than to emphasise however the NHS is changed by this, or any other government, the fact is, it is one of the largest public administrations left in Europe. It is complex, consumes a staggering amount of public money and employs an army of people with a kaleidoscope of skills. It is intricate, diverse and vital to our national interest. Therefore, how it is run is pivotal to its success and survival.

How else should this much loved institution be run other than in a businesslike way? The custodianship of public money demands standards of corporate governance that are part of the everyday of big business life. The vital, life saving work of the NHS demands quality standards and clinical governance that are to be found at the foundation of the zero defect environment of the best of successful businesses. The obligation to ensure all government departments work together in the common pursuit of 'wellness' demands intricate planning and strategy reaching the gold standard of the best that business can teach us. If the techniques of business are inescapable, then the language of business is inescapable too.

Business planning, whatever it's called, won't go away. The next section is devoted to business planning – no apology offered!

# Business Planning

# SECTION 4

## What about the business of business planning?

You'll have to do one sooner or later so here's the low down… Let's start with a couple of definitions.

## A business plan and a business case. What is the difference?

Business planning is a well-known concept, making a business case is less understood. The difference? Largely a matter of timing.

## The business plan

Typically, a business plan is written for a fixed period of time and plots the strategic direction of an organisation. Planning for a one year period is relatively straightforward. A plan for up to five years, in detail, with firm assumptions, needs care and attention to detail. Some say planning over such a long period, at a time of great change, is a waste of time. Unless you are Mystic Meg, no one can predict the future. However, we can make assumptions and develop the tactics and techniques to deal with what is ahead.

The longer the period a plan addresses, the greater the attention that has to be paid to the likely impact of factors from outside. That is why there is such emphasis on the SWOT analysis in the planning process – there are some exercises about SWOT earlier in the workbook.

Flexibility becomes a major consideration. For example, commissioning services over a three to five year period must allow for an annual review. Not just because funding is cash limited and demand difficult to predict, but changes in practice and new therapies will have to be accommodated. A plan that locks into a timeframe that doesn't allow for change, effectively locks out improvements that could deny patients the benefits of new technology.

## The business case

Making a business case is generally for the development of a new service or for the substantial re-development of an existing one. Making the case, or the justification, for a development.

Unlike the business plan that is usually linked to a planning cycle, the business case is developed as and when it is needed. However, for new developments involving new services, ensuring there is enough revenue in the system to pay for your wonderful new ideas means more planning, gathering support from the world and his wife and is often part of the planning cycle.

## Making the next bit work for you!

This next bit provides you with a series of checklists, questions and reminders to help cover the aspects needed to develop the business plan and case and produce a professional document.

The checklists are based on approaches in the professional, private and public sectors. Whilst the NHS is not a business, in the traditional sense of the word, it is moving towards ever greater efficiency by adopting some of the best practices common in business. Perhaps that's the third way!

Planning is a cornerstone of success. Focusing on the needs of 'customers' (a dirty word in the NHS, I know, but it does get you in the right frame of mind!), seeking out efficiencies and thoughtful planning are the keys to success for any business, public or private.

If you are ready to go ahead, scribble the answers to the questions on the page of the book – use it as a draft. Write on the pages of a book! No respect for the printed word!

# Assembling a business plan: flow chart

| Section 1 | Situation analysis | |
|---|---|---|
| | New information<br>National requirements etc. | |
| Understanding the environment in which the activity is to take place | **Key findings**<br>Observations from the environment and trends | |
| | **Opportunities and threats**<br>The effect of the 'environment'<br>Relative importance | |

| Section 2 | Success factors | Check capabilities. Can you do it with the skills available? |
|---|---|---|
| | Use opportunities and threats analysis to stimulate thinking on what is required | |
| Identifying the success factors | **Down-side analysis**<br>Anticipate problems and weaknesses | |

| Section 3 | SWOT | |
|---|---|---|
| | Summary of external and internal analysis | |
| Situation analysis<br>What can realistically be managed? | **Key issues**<br>Opportunities and threats that are realistic and based on your strengths and weaknesses | |

| Section 4 | Critical success factors | Double check forecasts are not over ambitious |
|---|---|---|
| | What you need to do... | |
| Performance expectations<br>What do you need to do?<br>What do we have to put in?<br>What can we expect to get out? | **Resource allocation**<br>Expenditure<br>Staff<br>Logistics | |

| Section 5<br>Key action planning | What to do next | Allocation of roles<br>Specific actions |
|---|---|---|
| | Who to see to get support<br>Specific actions<br>By when<br>By whom | |

| Section 6 | Review and check<br>Monitor milestones | |
|---|---|---|

## Let's give it a go: different strokes for different folks

### Who is the plan for?

The plan might be for a variety of interested parties. Just as books, magazines and newspapers take into account who their readership is, so must the planner. Who reads the plan means adjusting how you write the plan.

Is the plan for:

- people in your department to give them a sense of direction and clarity?

- your boss or a group of people who have the power to say 'yes' or 'no'?

- people who will 'invest' or fund the project or service?

- people who will use the service?

- people who will work in the service and run it?

- people who will give permission for the project to get underway?

- ...perhaps it will be a combination of all of them?

When you produce the plan put yourself in the shoes of the person who will read it and make the decisions to enable it to happen. Be honest with yourself. Does it make sense and can you deliver?

What will they need to get out of the plan to help them make a decision? Write your plan through the reader's eyes.

The plan must answer at least four questions:

1  what is your activity now?

2  are you competing for approval or resources? If so, how are you different (what makes you the best choice), *or* can you demonstrate you have satisfied the key requirements for approval?

3  what are your tactics, what do you need to do to win approval or resources, or turn your plan into a reality?

4  what are the benefits? Such as improvement in health gain or greater efficiency?

It is unlikely you will have all the information you need at your finger tips, to complete the plan.

- Whose support do you need to complete the plan?

- Who do you need to talk to, to gather the information that is required? Who are the other stakeholders?

- What does it mean in terms of their time and yours?

Matching diaries is never easy when folk are busy. Is your timescale realistic?

Before you plan your plan, plan the time it will take to assemble the detail.

Let's take it step by step...

## Step 1  The name of the organisation writing the plan?

If the plan is for a PCG then the name will probably already be in place. If the plan is for a department or a new project where the name will be different or new, think about how the name is to be selected?

- Will there be a competition?

- Will the name be based on geography, a focal point in the area?

- Will the name conflict with a name that is already in use?

- Is the name credible and will it stand the test of time?

- Does the name identify what you do?

- Is the name an ego trip for the organisation or will it mean something for or to the public?

## Exercise

 Describe how the name might be chosen. If the name is already chosen, is there 'buy-in' to the name? Do people like it, do they identify with it? Does it matter? Think about the plan you are about to write and ask if there is a title or a short phrase that would crystallise its purpose. Write it here:

## Step 2  Does the project have a home?

In the longer run, is the project likely to develop beyond 'the corner of a desk'?

## Exercise

• Is the project housed in appropriate accommodation?

• Is there a need to take into account the possibility of growth and a new home? What are the timescales?

• What are the practicalities of finding a new home?

• Are offices available?

• Does a planning consent have to be sought?

• What does that mean in terms of time?

• What about telephone lines and stationery and all that boring stuff?

## Step 3 Does the organisation have a mission statement to help focus everyone on the same goals?

Organisations are never what they seem. A delivery company does not just deliver parcels, they deliver our goods, in one piece, on time and without delays. A restaurant is not a restaurant, it is a quick snack, a romantic evening or a business lunch.

**Exercise**

Your mission statement:

## Step 4  Who is going to be responsible for writing the plan?

Organising the detail of the plan, collating the information and drafting takes time. Who is going to do it? Do they have a day job and are trying to fit this project in with everything else in their in-tray? Is it practical? Is the research phase resourced?

Consider what new people you will need to run and develop your project or plan, and allow lead time for recruiting, induction and training. Lead times for senior managers can run to two to three months.

Very few people really do hit the ground running. If you need to hire staff, remember that anyone who is any good will already be doing a good job for someone else. Allow time for them to disengage from their current employment and allow time for induction and settling in.

## Exercise

- What extra skills does the organisation need?
- Are there sufficient skills in the organisation?
- Is extra training required?
- Do the people have the time to deliver?
- Are you dumping responsibilities on willing shoulders that eventually will fail?

## Step 5 Demand

The concept of planning is relatively new, even to industry. It is a technique that is less than 50 years old. Only in recent years has it been adopted by the public sector and, probably, only a regular management tool in the NHS since the Thatcher reforms of the NHS in 1990.

Phrases, such as demand, never sat easily in the NHS dictionary. It is a word that is too close to the business community to be adopted readily by the NHS. Nevertheless, 'demand' or other phrases that indicate the extent to which services will be used, are a vital part of planning. If the plan is to underpin the development of a new service, establishing demand is fundamental. If the plan is in the context of a start-up organisation getting some clarity about what it is offering and how it is to do it, then 'demand' as part of the planning formulae is indispensable.

Don't overestimate demand and don't underestimate how hard it is to get a new idea off the ground.

## Exercise

For business cases, identify who is going to use the service and what evidence you have that the service will be used. Define, precisely, the services to be offered and show how you will let people know you are offering the service. Is the demand for the service seasonal, cyclical or constant? Finally, health is a high-tech business and today's good idea can easily be overtaken. Demonstrate how you will keep ahead of the game.

## Interlude: time for some finance stuff

Not all plans will need to have detailed financial information in them. Most do, but not all. The type of plan that does not need financial detail might be an introductory document, designed for internal use, that clarifies issues such as structure and who does what.

However, most plans will need some financial data to back them up. Here are the main headings that the financial detail will fall under:

### A balance sheet

This is an overall position statement setting out the value of the organisation, its assets, its income and expenditure.

### A 'profit and loss account'

Profit and loss is an expression commonly used in the business community and hardly needs a definition. In the NHS, where profits are not made, it is probably easier to think of it as income and expenditure. Profits might be seen as managing surpluses or losses on activity, manpower and finances.

### A cash-flow forecast

Cash flow is seen as the life blood of most business. Companies that trade at the margins of profitability can sometimes keep going, for longer than they should, because they have a positive, regular and healthy cash flow. It is also true that very profitable organisations have crashed because their cash flow has been poor and they have run out of money.

The public sector is fortunate in that it has a 'draw-down' arrangement with the Treasury and cash flow is not such an issue. The flow of cash through the organisation is a concern for directors of finance who need to know when they are likely to be called upon to make payments and when they are to expect receipts. All this gets turned on its head if there is an unexpected demand on services, such as in the winter months, and there is not enough cash in the system to pay the bills.

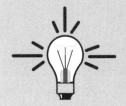

**THINK BOX**

Health is, increasingly, encouraged to work creatively with partners outside the NHS. Organisations such as social services and some others in the private and voluntary sector. If a project is to be joint funded, or to come from the newly 'pooled budget' arrangements with social services, think about timescales.

The public sector financial year runs April to March. Is that the same for everyone you are involved with? Are different accounting arrangements within different organisations likely to be a problem?

## Keeping up-to-date with what is happening

Make sure your plan allows for regular up-dates of the financial situation. Don't be shy about circulating budgets. People have got to know where they are – good or bad.

Regular reports are called management accounts. They should be produced regularly and consistently, in the same format so that it is easy to identify trends. They must be detailed enough to be interesting and helpful, but not so detailed as to be confusing.

Computer technology can be used to employ accounting packages that are capable of displaying complex information in graphical and simple to understand ways. Software is cheap and misunderstandings expensive. Graphs, bar charts and graphics can compare last month with this month and the year to date with targets – easy!

## Exercise

How financially literate are the people you work with? It's OK not to be an accountant! Honest! The important thing is that reports are regular and everyone who has responsibility understands what's going on. PCG Boards may not be entirely populated with people who feel comfortable with the numbers.

Develop a system for financial reporting that is accurate, not threatening to non-finance members and can be produced easily. What does technology have to offer?

## Step 6  Income and expenditure forecast

A PCG is forbidden by statute to make a 'loss', or in the language of the public sector, spend more than its allocation. So, unless you want an uncomfortable time with the Public Accounts Committee at the House of Commons, understand this next bit!

PCGs at Level 1 will have all the financial grunge taken care of by the health authority. Level 2 is a bit more exciting and there will be nominal budgets flying around that everyone will have fun 'nominally spending' or perhaps 'nominally saving'!

No matter, Levels 3 and 4 beckon where the hard, ugly world of hard, ugly cash lives. In the meantime, keeping an eye on what the finance experts at the health authority are doing is no bad thing.

Finance may be something you aren't 'doing' now, but you will have to. So make a start, here.

Start up projects using pump-priming funds, the sort that will require a business case, may legitimately not have their income matching their expenditure. The short-fall may be picked up elsewhere. Be careful to make realistic projections and if there is an excess of expenditure over income, don't hide it. The key is to be realistic.

Decide over what period you can realistically forecast in detail. In the world of business, high volume, high turnover activity is measured in weeks and months. Low volume, low turnover in months and years.

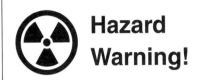

**Hazard Warning!**

Be sure to be realistic with projections and if there is an excess of expenditure over income, don't hide it. The key is to be realistic.

Think of a forecast as a photograph of how you see activity taking place. A careful picture of the detail up close and a snap of what the view might be from further away.

## Step 7  The income flow forecast

In business this would be called the cash-flow forecast – it's all the same. The forecast is simply a chronological list of expected expenditure deducted from anticipated income.

The calculation is done month by month, through the year. Include all expenditure and remember leases are not free – include them.

Here is an example of a cash-flow chart with some sample headings:

## Sample cash-flow chart (first year)

| Month | 1 | 2 | 3 | 4 | 5 | 6 | 7 | 8 | 9 | 10 | 11 | 12 |
|---|---|---|---|---|---|---|---|---|---|---|---|---|
| Total income | | | | | | | | | | | | |
| **Opening balance (A)** | | | | | | | | | | | | |
| Initial investment/grants etc | | | | | | | | | | | | |
| Income | | | | | | | | | | | | |
| Asset disposal | | | | | | | | | | | | |
| Interest on deposits | | | | | | | | | | | | |
| **Total income (B)** | | | | | | | | | | | | |
| Payments | | | | | | | | | | | | |
| Purchase of lease/property | | | | | | | | | | | | |
| Furniture/fittings | | | | | | | | | | | | |
| Vehicles | | | | | | | | | | | | |
| Materials | | | | | | | | | | | | |
| Employees wages, tax, NI | | | | | | | | | | | | |
| Training costs/conferences | | | | | | | | | | | | |
| Rent/rates | | | | | | | | | | | | |
| Fuel | | | | | | | | | | | | |
| Telephone | | | | | | | | | | | | |
| Post | | | | | | | | | | | | |
| Printing/stationery | | | | | | | | | | | | |
| Subscriptions/periodicals | | | | | | | | | | | | |
| Public meeting costs/promotion | | | | | | | | | | | | |
| Repairs/maintenance | | | | | | | | | | | | |
| Vehicle costs | | | | | | | | | | | | |
| Travel | | | | | | | | | | | | |
| Insurance | | | | | | | | | | | | |
| Professional fees | | | | | | | | | | | | |
| Loan/grant repayments | | | | | | | | | | | | |
| Bank charges | | | | | | | | | | | | |
| VAT | | | | | | | | | | | | |
| Other expenses | | | | | | | | | | | | |
| **TOTAL OUTGOING (C)** | | | | | | | | | | | | |
| Receipts, less payments for the month (D) (B − C = D) | | | | | | | | | | | | |
| Cash remaining in the PCG | | | | | | | | | | | | |

## Sample cash-flow forecast chart (years 2 & 3)

| Year/quarter | 2/1 | 2/2 | 2/3 | 2/4 | 3/1 | 3/2 | 3/3 | 3/4 |
|---|---|---|---|---|---|---|---|---|
| Receipts | | | | | | | | |
| **Opening balance (A)** | | | | | | | | |
| Initial investment/grants etc | | | | | | | | |
| Income | | | | | | | | |
| Asset disposal | | | | | | | | |
| Interest on deposits | | | | | | | | |
| **Total income (B)** | | | | | | | | |
| Payments | | | | | | | | |
| Purchase of lease/property | | | | | | | | |
| Furniture/fittings | | | | | | | | |
| Vehicles | | | | | | | | |
| Materials | | | | | | | | |
| Employees wages, tax, NI | | | | | | | | |
| Training costs/conferences | | | | | | | | |
| Rent/rates | | | | | | | | |
| Fuel | | | | | | | | |
| Telephone | | | | | | | | |
| Post | | | | | | | | |
| Printing/stationery | | | | | | | | |
| Subscriptions/periodicals | | | | | | | | |
| Public meeting costs/promotion | | | | | | | | |
| Repairs/maintenance | | | | | | | | |
| Vehicle costs | | | | | | | | |
| Travel | | | | | | | | |
| Insurance | | | | | | | | |
| Professional fees | | | | | | | | |
| Loan/grant repayments | | | | | | | | |
| Bank charges | | | | | | | | |
| VAT | | | | | | | | |
| Other expenses | | | | | | | | |
| **TOTAL PAYMENTS (C)** | | | | | | | | |
| Receipts, less payments for the year/quarter (D) (B – C = D) | | | | | | | | |
| Cash remaining in the PCG | | | | | | | | |

## Sample opening balance sheet

| *Liabilities* | *£* | *Assets* | *£* |
|---|---|---|---|
| Initial grants/loans | | Fixed assets | |
| Brought forward surplus | | Buildings | |
| | | Plant | |
| | | Furniture | |
| | | Vehicles | |
| | | Computers | |
| | | Equipment | |
| | | Other | |
| | | **TOTAL** | |
| Deferred liability | | Current assets | |
| Term loans | | Pharmacy | |
| **TOTAL** | | X-ray materials | |
| | | Other | |
| | | Cash | |
| Current liabilities | | | |
| Creditors | | | |
| Tax liability | | | |
| Bank overdraft | | | |
| **Total** | | | |

## Step 8  Capital equipment

If your plan envisages the acquisition of any capital equipment, you must detail what it is, and how its purchase is to be financed. Such items might include computers, fax machines and office furniture. A plan might concern the development of buildings or extensions to existing premises.

---

# Exercise

 List all the capital items (costing more than £300) required in the first three years; including (in each case), how it will be purchased – lease, loan, cash, rent etc.

| Capital item | Initial cost | Time of anticipated purchase | Method of payment | Completion of loan etc |
|---|---|---|---|---|
|  |  |  |  |  |
|  |  |  |  |  |
|  |  |  |  |  |

**Plus**

- What is the procurement process for new items? Are items to be researched and selected, or is a specification to be drawn up and bids invited? Who is going to do it and by when?

- Where is the line of accountability?

- Draw up a complete list of the equipment you will need to get you started. Consider how they will be financed.

## Step 9 Pharmacy, formulary and consumables

Add this step if there is a pharmacy element in the plan. How the pharmacy and arrangements for replenishing consumables are to be handled and how formulary decisions are to be arrived at.

- Group purchase?

- Who's in charge?

- Accountability?

- Decisions and methodology of adding new drugs to the formulary.

In business this would be 'stock control' and the same approach is good for PCGs and other public sector projects. Stock control is good discipline.

Too much stock (or consumables) and valuable money is tied up unnecessarily. Too little and you run the risk of running out of something vital.

Three words to remember about stock control: quantity, value, frequency.

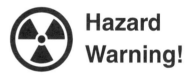 **Hazard Warning!**

Consider the impact of the Millennium Bug on your suppliers and their ability to deliver. If you don't know anything about the Millennium Bug, take my advice and stop living down a hole in the ground, try and get out more!

Consider re-order levels and lead time for replenishment and minimum levels it is safe to operate at.

High-tech devices often come with expensive consumables to make them work. Be sure to make realistic estimates about the frequency and costs involved.

## Step 10  Management information systems

Things can go wrong in every organisation, it is no great sin. The sin is not knowing that something has gone wrong!

A simple way to describe management information systems is 'keeping a finger on the pulse'. An organisation is very much like a living thing. Progress is measured by the day and progress from one day to the next can be very different. Sometimes the enterprise will be fit and healthy and at other times it could be a bit under the weather. Diagnosing a sick organisation is the job of managers – the organisation's doctor! To make a diagnosis you need a list of symptoms – they are called management reports.

Reports will include:

- cash flow
- income
- expenditure
- activity levels.

## Management accounts

### Sample headings

|  | Month 1 | Month 2 | Month 3 |
|---|---|---|---|
| *Employment costs* <br> Wages, salaries etc <br> Training |  |  |  |
| *Premises* <br> Rent <br> Rates/water |  |  |  |
| *Running costs* <br> Fuel <br> Telephone <br> Postage <br> Printing <br> Subscriptions <br> Vehicles |  |  |  |
| One off, start-up costs |  |  |  |
| Repairs <br> Insurance <br> Professional fees <br> Interest payments <br> Bank charges |  |  |  |
| Depreciation – vehicles <br> Depreciation – other assets |  |  |  |
| Other expenses |  |  |  |

## Step 11  Special factors

Will any special permissions need to be sought?

• Local authority – planning permission?

• County Council – licensing for nursing homes and the like?

• Fire Officer – fire certificates for buildings that the public have access to?

• Police – staff vetting for services to the vulnerable etc?

• What about employment legislation requirements?

• Shops and Factories and Offices Act?

• Disposal of waste.

---

**Exercise**

 If special permission is likely to be needed, establish how long it takes to obtain a consent. Some government and local government departments grind exceedingly slow!

---

## Step 12 Key decision dates

Think through all the stages that will take you to the first day of the operation of your plan (or new service). Buying equipment, finding premises, recruiting staff and the host of little jobs that make up the whole job done.

Sometimes it is easier to work back from a known starting date. The 'work back' approach is very useful, particularly when it reveals that to get to where you want to be in three months' time, you should have started four weeks earlier!

---

### Exercise

 Develop a schedule of key decision dates, working back from the end point and making some realistic decisions about timescales.

## Step 13 Can it work?

Now is the time for another SWOT analysis. This time for the plan.

Here's a reality check:

OK

1  Starting a new project is never easy. Is it a real team effort or is it in the hands of the odd enthusiast? Is the project sound enough to outlast the people who start it up?
2  Is technology involved? Do you really have the technical skills to make this work?
3  Is training required? Have you allowed time for training and for the cost of training?
4  Do you have the skills to administrate the project? How can you be sure the enthusiast won't run away with the idea, someone has to keep their feet on the ground and do the adding up!
5  Is the plan flexible enough to accommodate likely changes on the way?
6  Have you got the time to take another project on?
7  If you need to recruit, have you left time to get the staff?
8  Can you be sure the staff are available? Is there any kind of recruitment crisis in the professional sectors you will be relying on?
9  Is there wage inflation in the sector?
10  Are there any transport requirements for staff?
11  What's so special about this project?
12  Is there really a demand or is it just an expression of professional ego, or me-too-ism?
13  Are you sure that the service you are offering is supported by potential users?
14  Will you be prepared to modify what you are offering in the light of patient experience or demand?
15  Is this the right time to introduce this service?
16  Are developments in technology likely to overtake you?
17  Have you spoken with potential users of the services? What is their impression of what you want to do?
18  How will you keep up-to-date with developments and demand?
19  Can you rely on the suppliers of your kit or consumables?
20  Are you starting with pump-priming money? How can you be sure you will be able to fund the service in the medium/long term?
21  Have you got adequate management information systems in place to keep abreast of what is going on?
22  Is the project sufficiently managed by a professional who is not emotionally attached to the project?
23  Is there full commitment for the project from others, such as peers, Board members, other service providers?
24  Are any special permissions, licences or consents required? Can you get them in time?

How many ticks have you got? If there are any 'crosses' think carefully before getting underway. Sort the problems now, before you start.

## Exercise

 Evaluate the **s**trengths, **w**eaknesses, **o**pportunities and **t**hreats to the plan.

Can you do it? Now is the time to be ruthless and honest. Have you got the skills and talents available to make it all work?

# Glossary of terms

| | |
|---|---|
| Assets | Everything the organisation owns or is due to it. Fixed assets are buildings and plant. Intangible assets are things like 'good will'. |
| Balance sheet | A statement of what the organisation owes and what it is owed. And, the value of items it has disposed of. |
| Cash flow | Net income, together with non-cash charges such as depreciation and charges to reserves. |
| Depreciation | Money set aside against income to write off the cost of a capital item over its useful life. It is not a cash transaction, just a book-keeping entry. |
| Overhead cost | The total of indirect materials and wages and expense costs of the organisation. |
| Working capital | The difference between current assets and current liabilities. |

## Quick check

Have you?

…Got the process sorted out? Who will have overall responsibility for finalising the plan? If members of the team are contributing individual segments of the plan, is there a timetable for them to work to? Who's doing the checking, the reminding and the collating?

…Decided on the format of the presentation of the plan? Think about style. How do you plan to do the…

## Headings

And what is the length of the body copy? Keep it simple, avoid technical language and use:

• bullet points

• to emphasise

• important points.

Steer clear of *fancy type* faces, they are a pest to read. Use Times Roman for the text and **Ariel** for the headings and leave the fancy stuff to the designers of perfume packaging.

…Planned the pages? You should aim for something like this:

**Front page** (cover): nothing fancy, the more businesslike the better, avoid scans, pictures, clip art and cartoons. If you are using colour, use black for all the text and use colour sparingly. Except for graphs, don't use more than one other colour.

**Contents page**: for easy reference. Not everyone who sees your plan will want to read all of it. Make sure the contents page is comprehensive and accurate.

**Statement of Mission**: reproduce your mission statement and let readers see where you are coming from and show you've thought about it.

**Introduction** to the organisation. A brief pen portrait of the project, its location, the number of staff and so on. Try and give people a 'feel' for the organisation.

**Objectives** in publishing the plan. This is a detailed section on what the project intends to do and why.

**Action Plan** stating how you intend to achieve your objectives and the deadlines you intend to keep to.

**Detailed supporting information** such as financial statements and projections and technical documents.

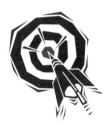

## On target?

How good is your plan?

Seven steps to evaluate a plan.

1 Is it realistic, can the project meet its financial obligations and formation criteria?

2 Where capital developments are involved, is there enough money in the system to pay for them and keep them running?

3 Does the plan fit in with national guidelines and local healthcare target imperatives (*Health of the Nation* and HImPs)? You do not exist in a vacuum. Indeed, health is, increasingly, set to play a role alongside other agencies in addressing disease.

4 Does it demonstrate complete control over all resources? Nothing left to chance and estimates (where absolutely necessary) based on conservative thinking.

5 Where applicable, thoroughly thought through strategies to deal with investment.

6 If any reliance is placed on non-NHS income (grants or staff for development from pharmaceutical companies, for example) what happens when the financing ends?

7 What is the sensitivity of the key assumptions, particularly around staff competencies? Are they realistic?

## Reporting systems

There are some basic questions you will need to answer.

If the project is set up in hierarchical groups (geographical, disease area or some other basis) it will be necessary to develop reporting systems to feed back. If knowing about the overall position of the organisation is dependent on drawing together from the reports of sub-groups, what are the arrangements for timely, accurate reporting? How is the project performing against budget? Will it run out of money before the end of the year?

Is there enough cash in the system to support the current level of activity, including staff and running costs?

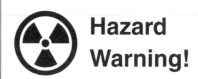

## Hazard Warning!

Is the information presented in a way that is understood by everyone? If people are not used to interpreting financial information, create an environment where it is OK for them to say so, without feeling foolish. No one should be put in a position where they don't understand and can't see problems looming up.

To answer these questions make sure:

- You have the information you want, presented in a way so you can understand it. It is no good a key player announcing, 'Oh, I didn't understand the financial position'.

- Ensure that the timetable for reporting is agreed and stuck to. Do not accept any excuses such as, 'The information wasn't available because there wasn't time'. Timeliness is more important than micrometer accuracy. If an army marches on its stomach, an organisation moves on its information systems.

## The golden rules of financial information

Current information should be compared against budgets. Is the project doing what it thought it would be doing. If not, why not?

- Is the information presented in a way that is understood by everyone? If people are not used to interpreting financial information, create an environment where it is OK for them to say so, without feeling foolish.

- Is the information being compared over the same period of time? If the information cycle is monthly make sure it stays that way, otherwise comparisons are meaningless.

- Make sure all the staff are aware of the budget position. If staff at the coal face know the problems they can help to dig the coal to get you out of a mess.

- Insist the budget is planned for the year ahead, not cobbled together half-way through the year.

- Do not accept that last year's budget will be the same next year. Always insist on zero budgeting, i.e. starting with a blank sheet of paper and assembling the budget from scratch.

- Don't get bogged down in unnecessary complications, with cross-department recharging and so-on.

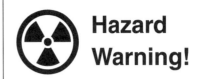

**Hazard Warning!**

Be on the look-out for shared costs, recharges, internal cost centres, departmental costs, nominal entries for repairs maintenance and services when they should be the real costs, or are duplicated costs.

## Getting a feel for what is going on

Newcomers may find an established organisation a mystery. New organisations are a mystery for everyone! Developing management controls is all part of keeping up with what the organisation is achieving and to ensure that it is on course.

## Congratulations on getting this far! Well done, have a coffee, or something stronger!

By now you should have thought about all the issues and collected all the information you need to be able to put together a plan under the following headings:

Yup, done it

1  The name of the project.

2  The location.

3  The Mission or nature of the project.

4  The people who will deliver it, their skills and talents.

5  A rationale about why the service or development is needed (demand).

6  How it is to be funded, both in start-up and ongoing.

7  The income stream (cash flow).

8  A list of the capital items you will need and how they are to be funded.

9  A statement of policy about stock or consumable items and how they are to be funded.

10  The sources of start-up capital, loans, grants, bids and so on.

11  How you will keep up-to-date with the progress of the project (management accounts).

12  Special factors that might include training, licences, permission.

13  An overall action plan setting out key target dates and contingencies.

# SECTION 5

## Making it stick

So, you've finished the plan. Everyone has admired your work, patted you on the back and said well done. Time to put your feet up and drink a cup of coffee?

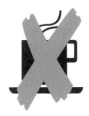

No, sorry, there's more to do. Planning is not a one off job, the document to be filed and forgotten. You are planning for the future and your next task is to see how the plan is working. Your plan might be for a period of years, or it might be for the duration of a specific project, either way you have to monitor events against the plan, to see if it is delivering.

## Monitoring success

You need to think about performance indicators to measure the plan against, holding regular meetings with the people implementing the plan and devising a method of measuring that objectives are being met.

## Exercise

Look at your plan and extract from it factors that can be used to monitor performance and success. Think of these as benchmarks that can be identified and become a tangible way of ensuring you are on track.

## Exercise

• Devise a meeting timetable that is frequent enough to keep in touch with progress, but not so frequent as to become a routine that everyone ignores.

• Who should attend the meetings.

• Does everyone involved have to attend all the meetings, all of the time?

# Exercise

How will you reappraise your plan?

Devise a system to:

- measure the organisation's performance against its mission and values

- ensure it is meeting its targets

- measure what is really happening against what you planned should be happening

- revisit financial forecasts.

If time reveals the plan is in some way flawed, what processes will you use to revise the plan and keep the agreement of everyone involved in the plan's successful delivery?

# Exercise

 Even the best laid plans of mice and men can be set to nought!

We can't quite recall which particular great person first said that but whoever it was, they are right. Expect the unexpected is the message. As part of the pre-planning process you will have conducted a SWOT analysis. The threats to the plan will have been the subject of careful evaluation and thought. However, the NHS is a special beast and inhabits an unpredictable world.

Although government appears willing to plan over a longer timescale than the traditional year-on-year approach, there is still the potential for external factors impacting on the best laid plans of mice and men.

A down-turn in the economy could mean a pressure on the NHS from the Treasury to make annual savings of 4% instead of 3%. The head count may become the subject of political interest and the 'men in grey suits' argument may be resurrected. 'Cut management numbers' is a familiar and easy cry from the safety of the backbenches in the House of Commons.

Think again about 'threats' and reconsider your plan. Don't unpick the plan if you have taken all reasonable factors into account. However, look at the plan in the context of what a contingency plan might look like, in the event of the wheels coming off somewhere else and the likely impact for you:

# SECTION 6

## Boxes in the attic

### Looking for ideas?

There's stuff lying around all over the place! None of it is rocket science and most of it has been lying around in boxes for years. A great man once said, 'there's no such thing as a new idea, just old ideas in new clothes'. Cynical but true… Here are some ideas.

Looking for thoughts on shaping your HImP? You need a health needs assessment. In other words find out what's important and what could be tackled. Only you can find out what is important in your area, the health issues that really need to be tackled. What's the best way to do it? Easy…

 Sit down, over a cup of coffee, with a health visitor and a district nurse. You'll find out all you need to know. In fact, why not organise a half-day seminar for health visitors and district nurses for them to talk about the health needs in your area – you'll be surprised the story they have to tell! That should give you some good ideas.

### What else?

Do you know the one about the motorist who got lost?

He stopped and asked directions from a vicar. 'Well' said his reverence, 'drive down here to St Michael's and turn right, go left at St Luke's and it's the third on the left past the convent'. The driver got confused and asked for the same directions from a publican. 'Ah' said the publican, 'drive down the road 'till you see the Dog and

Duck and turn right, go left at the Crown and Cushion and it's just across the road from the Prince of Wales'.

Two answers that got to the same conclusion – from two perspectives. Who we are and what we do affects how we see things. Health needs assessments must come from more than one perspective. Generally, there are three players.

**Epidemiologists**, **professionals** (not just clinical professionals but ones outside health too) and the **punters** (that's not just patients, users and carers, but the general public as well). They will all have a different perspective on just about every facet of healthcare. All equally valid and more often than not, equally persuasive. HImPs give us, now, the opportunity to work together and look at some of the causes of ill health by thinking outside the box. Seeing each other's point of view and working with other professionals. Let's look at a health related issue that crosses the boundary between primary care, secondary care, the voluntary sector and social care. Let's, just for an example, have a look at booze!

Most health authorities will spend a tidy sum on alcohol services and substance misuse clinics. Social services will probably have a budget for dealing with the problem, too. Is it an issue for you and could the money being spent now, be better spent if all the agencies involved worked together?

What should the aim be? Spend less on the service, spend more on the service or get better value for the money you are spending now?

Is all booze harmful? Don't some docs tell us a glass of whisky a day does the ticker good? Perspectives are a real pain aren't they? Ask the epidemiologist. He or she will be able to tell you interesting stuff like:

- the number of drunks messing up the A&E every Saturday night

- the number of patients that turn up in A&E with a bump on the head, or some other assault, having been bashed by someone who has had too much to drink

- the number of people who cannot control their drinking and are in psychiatric care

- deaths from booze related cancers.

…and if you push them, they will also be able to put their hands on the numbers for:

- convictions for drink driving

- traffic accidents where alcohol is a determinant

- drink related criminal damage.

…ask them again and they might even be able to get some numbers on child abuse and marital problems that are thought to be drink related. If you stop and think about it there are scores of professionals and organisations who deal with the problems that are the by-product of alcohol.

Ask the punters about alcohol and my guess is that senior citizens will talk about being put off shopping by youngsters drinking cans of beer in the town centre and the youngsters will tell you about drunks in clubs, getting drunk and getting pregnant. Whoever you ask will have their own perspective and they will all be right!

So, what's realistic?

• Banning all drinking?

• Get the police to chase the drunks out of the town centre?

• Do something about the 'binge-boozers' who do the damage on Friday and Saturday nights?

• Encourage people to limit their drinking to the recommended levels? The so called 'safe' levels.

• Work with people who are alcohol dependent?

Time for another coffee and 'think'. Look at the list. Before HImPs no one in health had a hope in hell of addressing the whole list. The conventional approach would have been to concentrate on one sector and settle for that. Now, we might just be able to have a go at it all! We can work with the Borough Council and the Chamber of Trade, to introduce local by-laws banning drinking in the town centre; get the police to target their shifts to focus on the worst nights of the week and sort out public order issues; work with the school and clubs to encourage the youngsters to treat drink with respect; work with employers to reduce alcohol related absences on Monday mornings; work with GPs to make the morning after pill available; work with pubs and clubs to get more condom machines installed. All that and not a mention of healthcare – but it is all healthcare, isn't it? Suddenly, it is all realistic! We can have a go at much more than just health. Can we make a list of all the things we could do, together, to address inappropriate use of alcohol?

Who would do it?

How?

- Define what we mean by sensible limits for different groups

- Discourage binge-boozing

- Change the patterns of drinking to reduce:

    - crime

    - traffic accidents

    - unwanted pregnancies

    - wilful damage

    - domestic violence

- Extend drinking hours

- Better bus service, taxis etc

- Re-roster police to meet peak demand for public order issues

- Availability of emergency contraception

- Examine the link between how to change attitude and how to change behaviour

- Evaluate services across primary and secondary care – can anything be redesigned? Must they be medical services or can they be social care-led.

- What can Alcoholics Anonymous, Drink Wise or Relate add?

OK, your turn! What do you want in your HImP? What are the issues?

---

## Exercise

 Devise a programme to establish a list of issues that might be included in your HImP.

Now consider how the list could be evaluated.

---

## Exercise

 What other agencies can be involved?

What is more important, the number of agencies or the outcome of the HImP?

## Exercise

 Most likely, other agencies and organisations will not be used to joint working in this way. This is grown-up joined-up stuff! How will you approach them? How will you get them on board? Did the selection of the HImP target involve them? What will it take to get them 'signed-up' to the idea?

## Exercise

 Does the HImP target involve budgetary expenditure or the shift of resources? If other agencies are involved, what is their budgetary cycle? Does it impact on the success of the scheme? Are you dealing with groups who can OK a budget? Local authorities may have to go back to their members and other services may have procedures and authorisations to go through. Can the objective be delivered in the planned operation year or will it have to run into the next financial year?

# Exercise

Who should lead the process? Health is the lead agency but does the project have to be led by a health person? What are the advantages of shifting the leadership outside health?

# Exercise

How will you know if you are successful? Design the evaluation criteria and a schedule for checking you are on target.